Grandma's Guide to Healthy Eating on a Budget

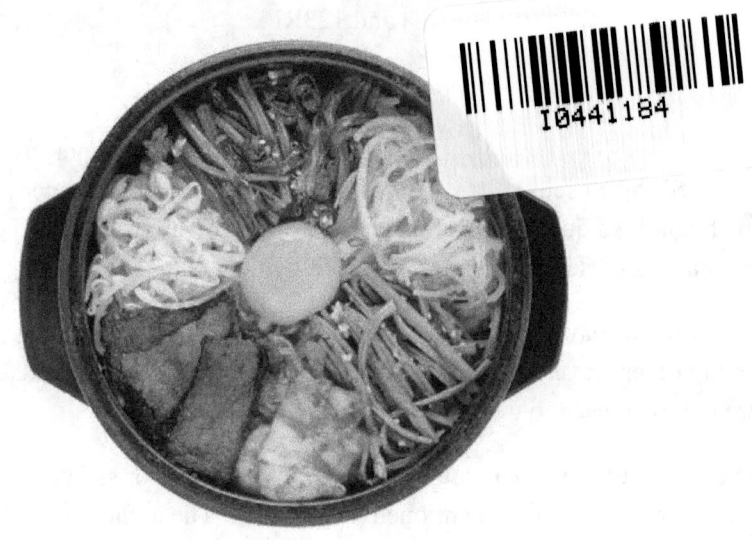

Healthy Old-Time and Traditional Recipes From All Over The World

Grandma Series

Dueep J. Singh

Mendon Cottage Books

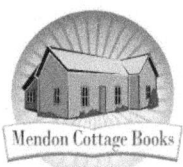

JD-Biz Publishing

Disclaimer

The information is this book is provided for informational purposes only. It is not intended to be used and medical advice or a substitute for proper medical treatment by a qualified health care provider. The information is believed to be accurate as presented based on research by the author.

The contents have not been evaluated by the U.S. Food and Drug Administration or any other Government or Health Organization and the contents in this book are not to be used to treat cure or prevent disease.

The author or publisher is not responsible for the use or safety of any diet, procedure or treatment mentioned in this book. The author or publisher is not responsible for errors or omissions that may exist.

Warning

The Book is for informational purposes only and before taking on any diet, treatment or medical procedure, it is recommended to consult with your primary health care provider.

Check out some of the other Healthy Gardening Series books at Amazon.com

Gardening Series on Amazon

Check out some of the other Health Learning Series books at Amazon.com

Health Learning Series on Amazon

Table of Contents

Introduction

We are at the beginning of a new era in food. If grandma had the financial resources, she made sure that her table was stocked with lots and lots of food, starting with soup, meat, vegetables, fruit and sweetmeats. A more frugal grandma would look at the limited ingredients in her garden, and in her kitchen and use her creativity to make a delicious meal as often as she could to feed her hungry brood.

Cooking was an art, in olden days, especially when traditional cooks knew all about the effect of different foods on your body and system.

In Korea and in many parts of the East, including China, the Royal family had special cooks who were half doctors themselves. They knew all about the internal system of each and every member of the royal family, and used special ingredients and cooking methods in order to keep their systems working properly and in a healthy manner. That is when the art of cooking was at its zenith; cooking to keep healthy and eating nutritious food.

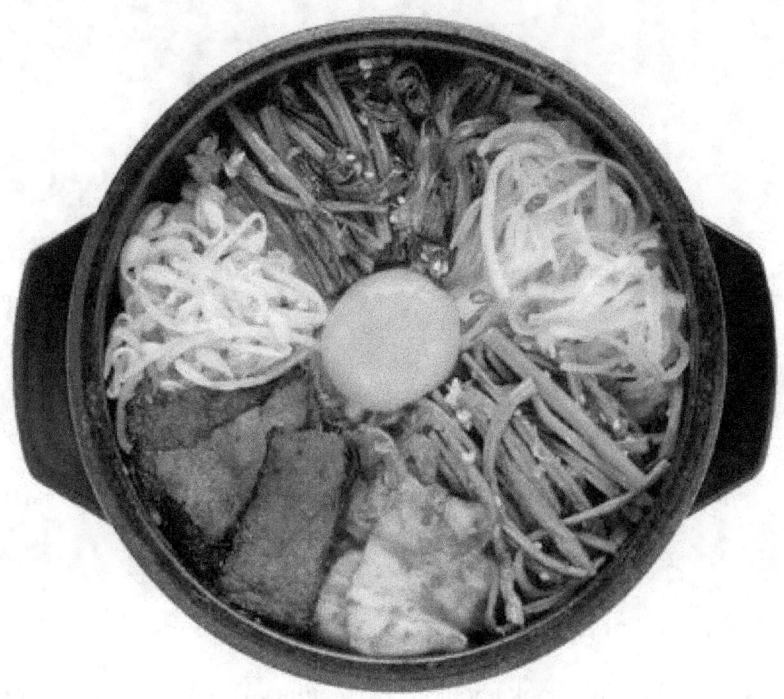

This is an example of traditional and ancient Korean healthy cooking – Bibimbap.

Thanks to that tradition which began to be followed all over the world through the centuries, the 21st century health-conscious cook has suddenly grown aware of what is good for his health and what is bad – what is too much to eat and why one should eat less.

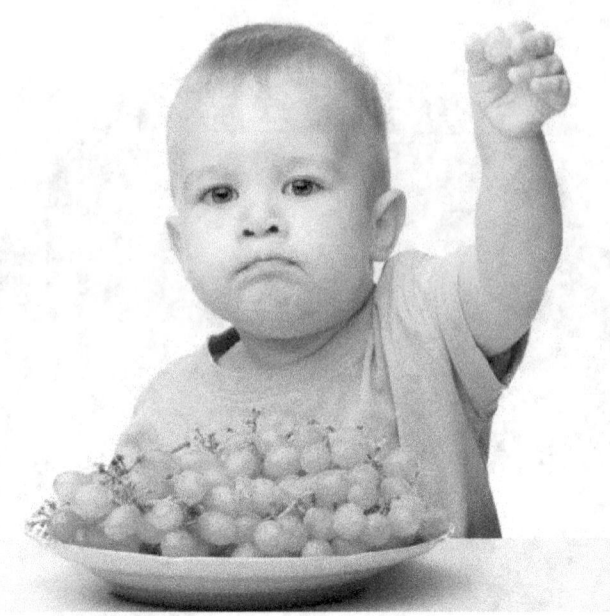

Every bit counts- but in moderation.

I remember reading in a book about an 18th-century fishing village, where the girls were extremely beautiful. One of these girls recounted her life to her grandchildren in these words. "Food was scarce in our village, and all that was available was given to the boys, because they had to go fishing. We girls got what was left and that is why we had thin slim forms and clear skin. That was good for us in the long run, I believe."

This may seem rather horrific to us, especially in a world of lessening gender prejudice against sons and daughters, but take into view, the fact that never has the world had so much food available to it than in the 20th and 21st century, it should not be surprising that our eating patterns changed drastically.

With so much food available to us, and in such large quantities, most of us ate whatever we could get, and whenever we go to get it, without bothering much about fitness. But fitness came naturally in grandma's time, when a sedentary lifestyle was anathema. Everybody worked from dawn to dusk and hard. And they ate like hungry wolves. But they never over-ate, because often, there was not so much food on the table and also, the work done throughout the day, burnt up all that extra layer of fat.

Many of these recipes given in the book are old favorites, especially those which may have disappeared from your table for a while, but which are going to come back time and time again, when more people begin to believe in healthy eating. Other recipes of traditional dishes have come from other countries where fitness is the rule, not the exception.

Many of the recipes being used in grandma's time, – and even before her time – were old family favorites that had been handed down through three or more generations.

Not only were they tested and proven and eaten regularly, they were for the most part, simple and yet unusual. In nearly all of them, the only ingredients needed were basic items which grandma kept on hand at all times.

These Budget Recipes, which include old-time recipes from grandma's cookbooks will also give you a good range of delicious recipes which you are going to enjoy preparing because they are so easy on your purse. You may also want to use leftovers to prepare new recipes, taking into consideration every ingredient you have used and giving you the most for your dollar.

Old-Style Eating Versus New Style Eating

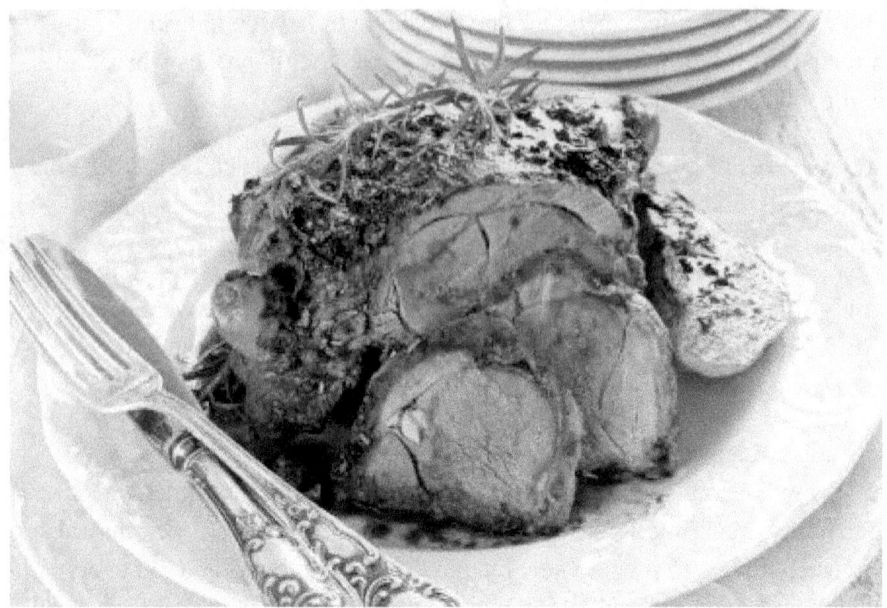

 Old-style eating and very good it can be was the traditional and heavy three-course lunch. New style eating is a larger collection of various dishes from which you choose small amounts to eat. Why has this change come about?

 Obesity is a growing concern among health-conscious people in the West, and eating trends recommend a time-tested eating rule – it makes sense to eat less. I was laughing on this point at a gathering of friends, where my American friend had taken three heaped tablespoons of one of the dishes he liked, while my French friend had more self-control and had taken one teeny-weeny teaspoon.

 When I asked François to spoil himself and take at least one more teaspoon – grinning all the while – he said that he was more concerned about enjoying the taste and texture. If he wanted more, he would take more. He did not want to overburden his plate at the first instance itself.

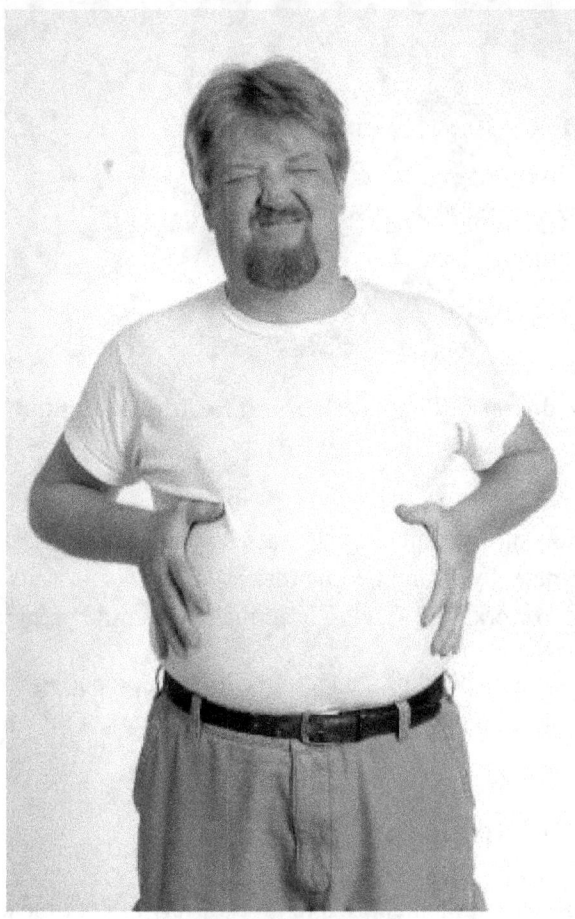

Too much overeating…

We pretended not to look at our overburdened plates because let us face it, when there is lots of food, we like a full plate. And that leads to overeating.

Small tempting dishes instead of one large main dish of meat and two vegetables is soon going to become the eating tradition of the West.

But, you say that you are so busy and you really do not have the time to make so many items. It is much better to stick to one dish cooking away slowly and ready in time when you come back from the office. Or better still, you intend to stick to that convenience food, you picked up while coming back home, at the delicatessen on the corner of the street in which you just need to add some water and you have a ready-made meal.

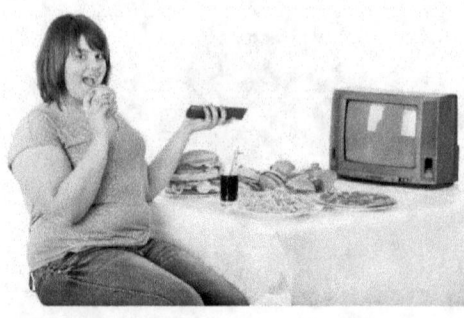

We do not bother much about healthy eating today.

This saves you lots of time but are you really eating healthy? Fast meals is partly due to a demand by young people for casual snacks. It is also due to more women going out to work, and serving food that needs little preparation.

Grandma did not mind spending hours in the kitchen preparing food. However, 21st-century sensible eating should be more oriented in a combination of heavy flavors and textures.

Tips For Healthy Food Serving

Here are some easy to implement tips to give variety to your meals.

Small portions made tempting – serve a variety of flavors and textures with plain boiled rice for an attractive Chinese or Spanish style meal.

Put spice into your meals – try out the Korean, Malaysian and Indian way of cooking with seasonings and spices. Fresh herbs also do wonders to an otherwise bland dish.

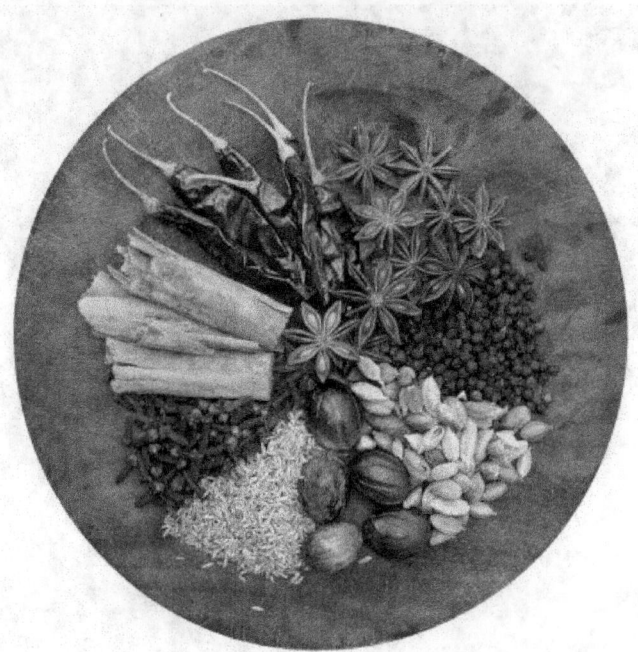

Eat less meat – more meat means more calories. If you cannot do without deep-fried onions, potato chips and meat steak, It means that you are adding 1889 cal to your calorie count with every meal.

Fast food – the good and the bad – do not eat chips with your hamburger. Instead, choose salad. Salt beef sandwich salad is a good meal, but the Sundaes should only be a rare treat.

Stir frying in a Wok- when grandma tossed in a large number of articles in her wok, and made a literal story, with crunchy vegetables, and only a little meat, she was emulating traditional Japanese meals. You can do that for a healthy meal.

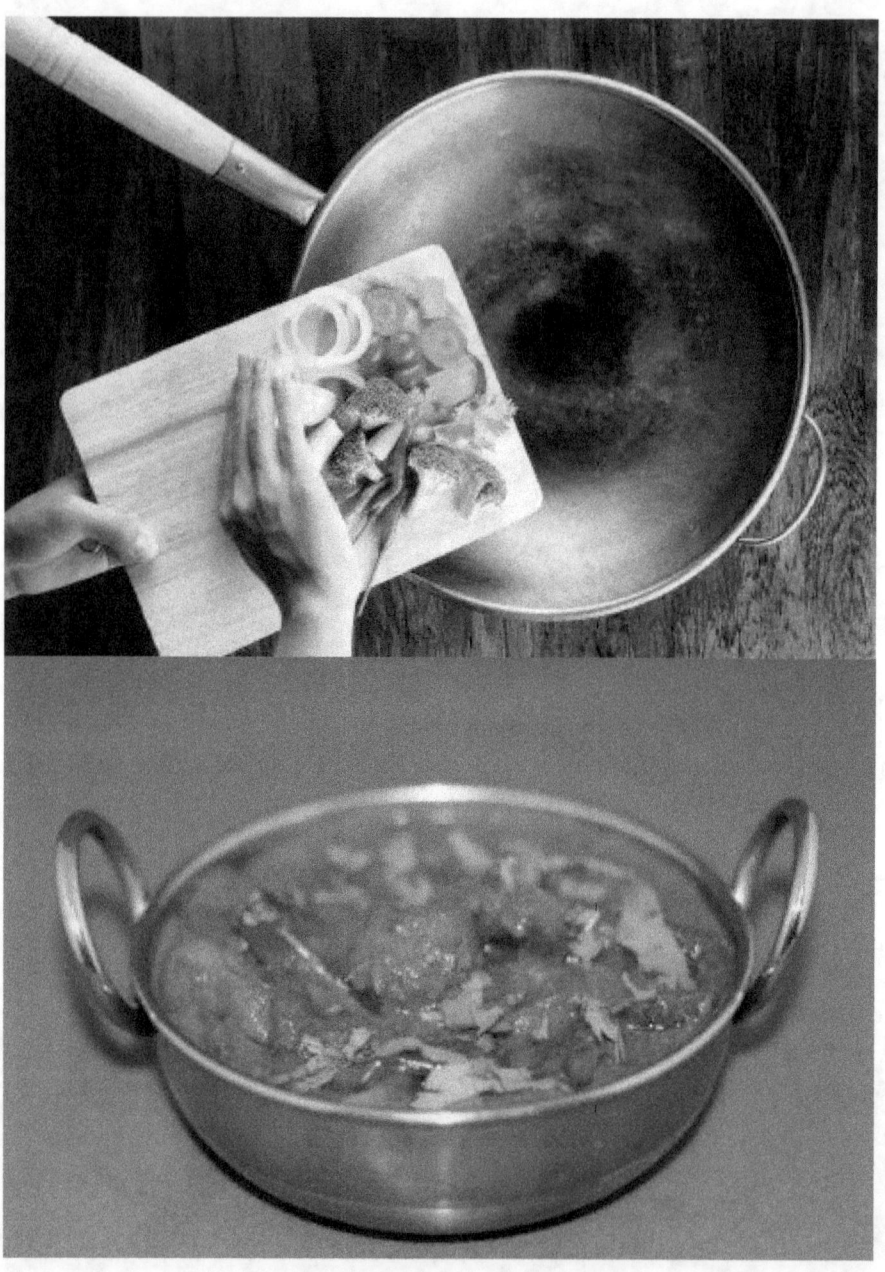

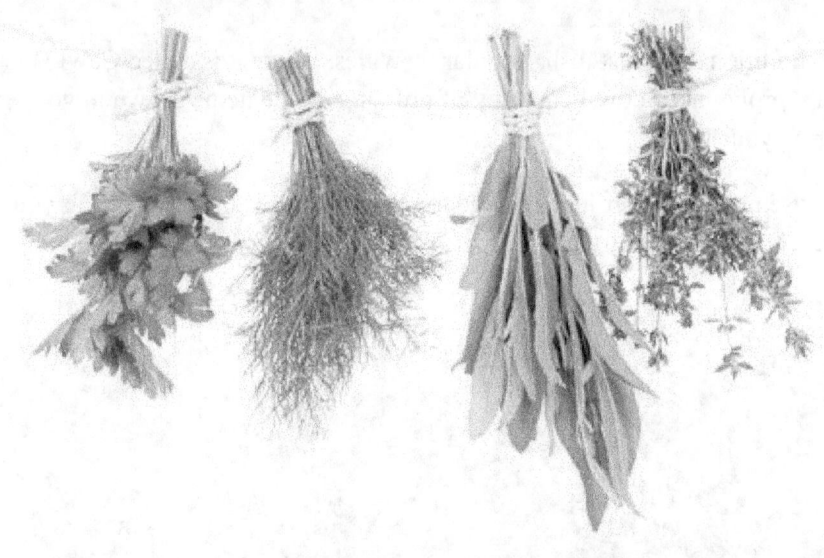

Use herbs as often as possible.

Harvest Stew

This is a traditional harvest dish, popular in Wales, where it is called Cawl Cynhaeaf – pronounced cow-l cun- hay-af utilizing all the items grown in your garden or on your farm.

You can use meat left over in the fridge to make this stew, but I am giving you the ingredients for six hungry people.

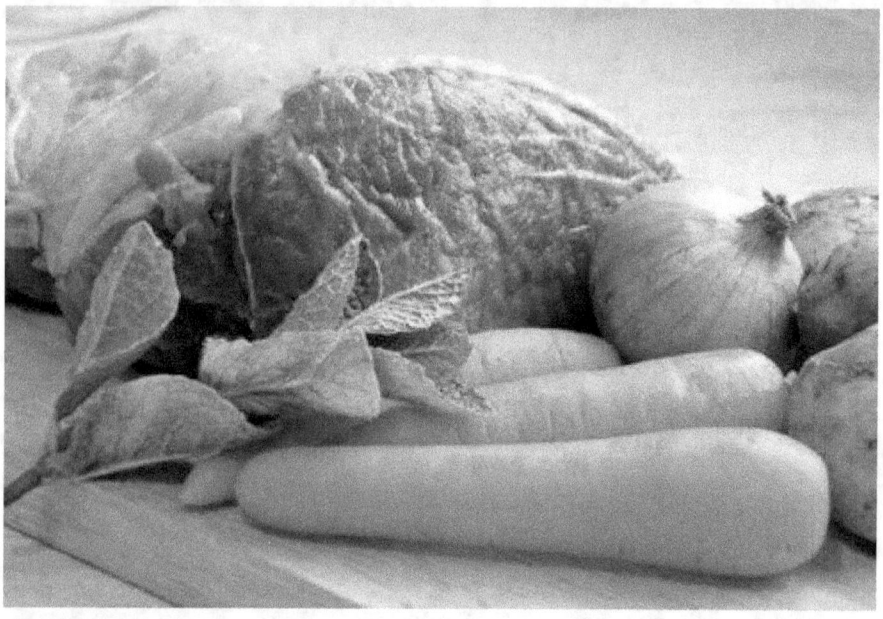

All available vegetables along with meat can make delicious harvest stew throughout the year.

2 pounds of stewing steak, cubed.

A little oil.
Two level teaspoons flour – grandma used unrefined flour, so you are going to do the same.
1 pound smoked back bacon – cubed. [This harvest stew is nutritious and delicious, and it is going to keep well in the fridge, so once you make it, you can heat it up as often as possible. Children love it and do not mind the

vegetables, because they are so busy picking out the meat pieces and chomping on them!]

1 ½ pints water.

My friend Gwen told me that her grandmother added half a pint of beer to give the stew more body, but I could add stout if I wished.

2 pounds of mixed seasonal vegetables – carrots, onions, leeks, potatoes, parsnips, cabbage, or any other vegetable prepared and cut into bite sized pieces.

A good range. Each of chopped marjoram, thyme and any other spicy like.

A few sprigs of rosemary. Seasoning as you wish, including salt and pepper.

Peel and chop or slice the vegetables. Any mixture is going to do, but leeks are both traditional and attractive.

The harvest stew is thickened with the flour. Traditionally, wholemeal stoneground flour with the bran still in was used, so if you can find that flour anywhere, you are going to notice the nutty and delicious flavor.

The dark beer, or even stout gives a good flavor to the stew. It also deepens the rich dark brown color.

A pinch of herbs, and the seasoning gives this stew that extra delicious zest, tang and flavor.

Fry the meat in a little oil to brown. Stir in the flour and cook, stirring, for two – three minutes. Gradually stir in the water and beer. Now add the other ingredients except for the potatoes and Leeks and bring to a boil. Leave to simmer, covered, for 1 ½ hours for that rich meat and vegetables taste. Now add potatoes and leeks, reserving a little shredded raw leek for garnishing.

Continue cooking for 15 to 20 minutes until all the vegetables are tender. Serve garnished with the reserved raw shredded leek.

When I made this dish for my father, he scoffed and said that he had eaten it in America – when he was living with a family on a farm. This was thanks to the American government's happy idea of showing their "guests" from India the taste of real America.

The lady of the house was really happy with father who loved eating everything put before him, and then praising it, because it reminded him so much of every mother's cooking all over the world – East or West!

So one day when he said that this stew could be improved by adding a little bit of fresh milk, she said, well, yes and did that in the last 15 minutes of cooking. The milk curdled, naturally, and the rest of the family blinked when the familiar dish was served before them with chunks of white. Now what was that? That was milk. When the giggling stopped, they found that the milk – even in its curdled form – improved the stew considerably.

That weekend, when Mrs. Bell was cooking the harvest stew father was there in the kitchen, mixing up the flour with the milk before putting it into the meat. So consider this to be Indian – Welsh – American harvest stew, eaten globally for those who are on a budget, enjoy good food and like to eat healthy, nourishing dishes.

. Mrs. Bell was astonished to hear that meat eating is not usually a common practice in the East, even though father was an omnivorous epicure.

That was when eating patterns were set out millenniums ago, where herbs and vegetables were a better food choice than going hunting in the jungle for fresh meat.

So here we start on the best choice of more international flavors and textures, with –

Fish With Tomato

One onion, finely chopped
2 tablespoons full of salt.
Half a pound of fresh fish fillets, cut into small pieces
Six large, organically grown tomatoes.
Garlic salt and black pepper to taste.

Fry the onion in the oil until transparent. Add the fish and cook for two – three minutes, and then add tomatoes and seasoning. Simmer for about five minutes until the fish is cooked through and the liquid has reduced.

Spinach salad

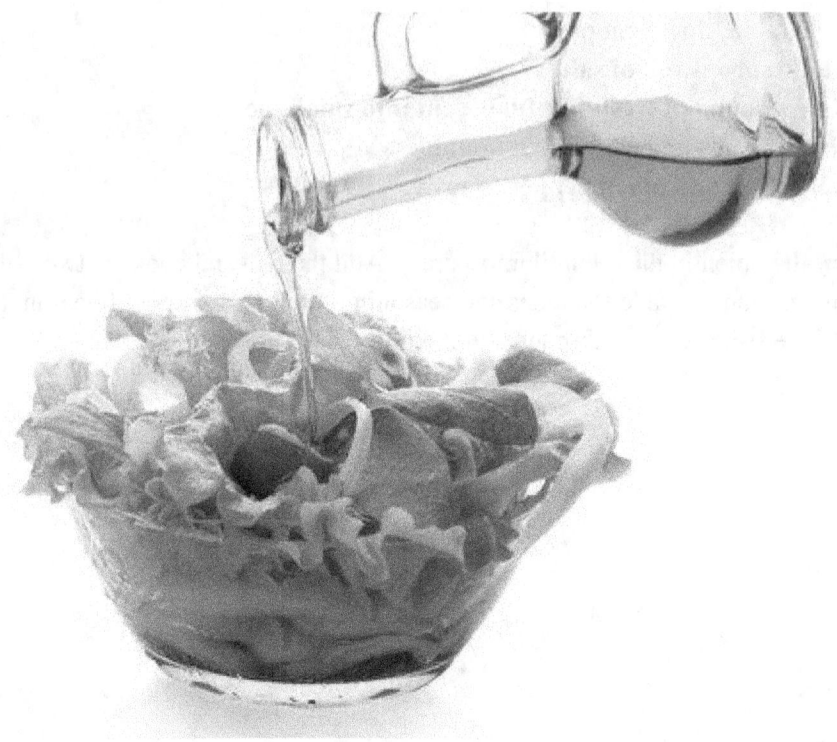

Toss about 1 ½ pounds of well washed spinach leaves in your favorite salad dressing and serve. I also add some boiled eggs, and some potatoes to this mixture.

You may also want to try out this version of spinach salad, which serves four – six.

4 ounces streaky bacon, chopped, half a pound of fresh spinach, half a pint of French dressing, seasoned with fresh herbs, 4 ounces of white Stilton cheese.

Fry the bacon until crisp. Wash and dry the spinach. Tear into shreds. Do not cut unless you have extended steel knife. Toss in the dressing. Crumble the Stilton and bacon over the spinach. Toss and serve immediately.

As spinach needs picking almost as soon as it is fully grown, and does not keep well, you may wish to freeze some now for later in the year. This can be washed and frozen uncooked, tightly packed in polythene bags. This is going to keep for three months. Or you can blanch for minimum time, squeeze out the excess water and freeze in the leaves or shredded, or puréed. I normally add a quarter teaspoonful of salt, before I blanch these leaves to preserve while freezing.

Traditional Salad Recipe

When I was making up the spinach salad recipe that reminded me of one of my favorite recipes in literature given to the writer of the Ingoldsby legends – the Rev. Barham.

Here it is –

A RECEIPT FOR SALAD

Two large potatoes passed through kitchen sieve,

Unwonted softness to the salad give;

Of ardent mustard add a single spoon,

Distrust the condiment which bites so soon;

But deem it not, thou man of herbs, a fault

To add a double quantity of salt;

Three times the spoon with oil of Lucca crown,

And once with vinegar, procured from town,

True flavour needs it, and your poet begs

The pounded yellow of two well-boiled eggs;

Let onion atoms lurk within the bowl,

And, scarce suspected, animate the whole;

And, lastly, on the flavored compound toss

A magic teaspoon of anchovy sauce.

Then, though green turtle fail, though venison's tough,

And ham and turkey are not boiled enough,

Serenely full, the epicure may say,--

'Fate cannot harm me, -- I have dined to-day.'

N.B.-- As this salad is the result of great experience and reflection, it is to be hoped young salad-makers will not attempt any improvements upon it.

This recipe was sent to him by someone unknown, who did not sign her/his name on the letter. But like the writer said, absolutely no one can improve on this delicious and tasty salad. Oil of Lucca is, of course Olive oil.

Beef in Ginger

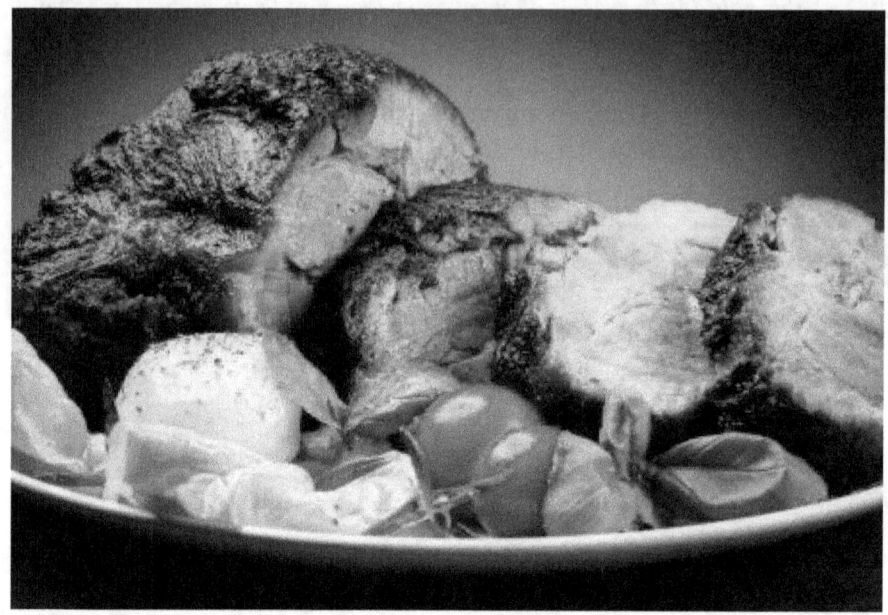

Beef, especially roasted with vegetables is healthy and economical

I am a great eater of beef, and I believe that does harm to my wit. Shakespeare had Sir Andrew Aguecheek saying this in Twelfth Night. That was because at that time a stupid person was called beef witted!

Nevertheless, veal and beef are healthy and proteinaceous additions on your table, so try this delicious dish.

This is going to serve five – six people.

Three large onions, peeled
Half a pint of beef stock
Half a pint brown ale.
1 ½ inches fresh root ginger
1 pound sirloin beef steak cubed
One level tablespoon full of corn flour, blended 2 tablespoons full of water.
Half a cucumber.
One clove of garlic.
Seasoning to taste and any other herbs you want added here.

Simmer the onions in the stock and the ale for fifteen minutes. Cut the cucumber into 2 inches lengths and add to the pan with finely chopped ginger, crushed garlic, seasoning and meat.

Simmer for 20 to 35 minutes. Stir in the corn flour, bring to a boil, and simmer for one – two minutes, stirring continuously.

Spiced Chicken Wings

Brush **twelve chicken wings with your choice of herbs and sweet pickle. Then grill. I like to marinate the wings beforehand in a mixture of yogurt, clove of garlic, paprika, salt, pepper and herbs.**

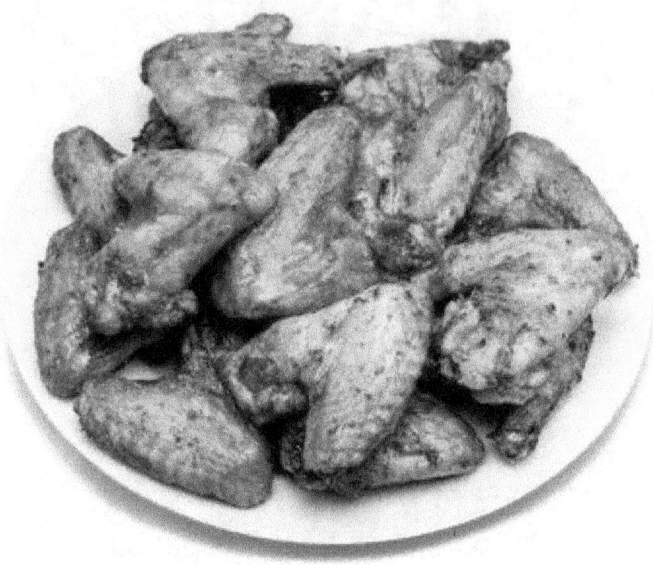

We can learn a lot from the Japanese and Chinese cuisines, when it comes to presenting a variety of foods in an attractive way. These dishes are served with just one small bowl of plain boiled rice. Not only do they look good, but they taste good.

Mixed Vegetables

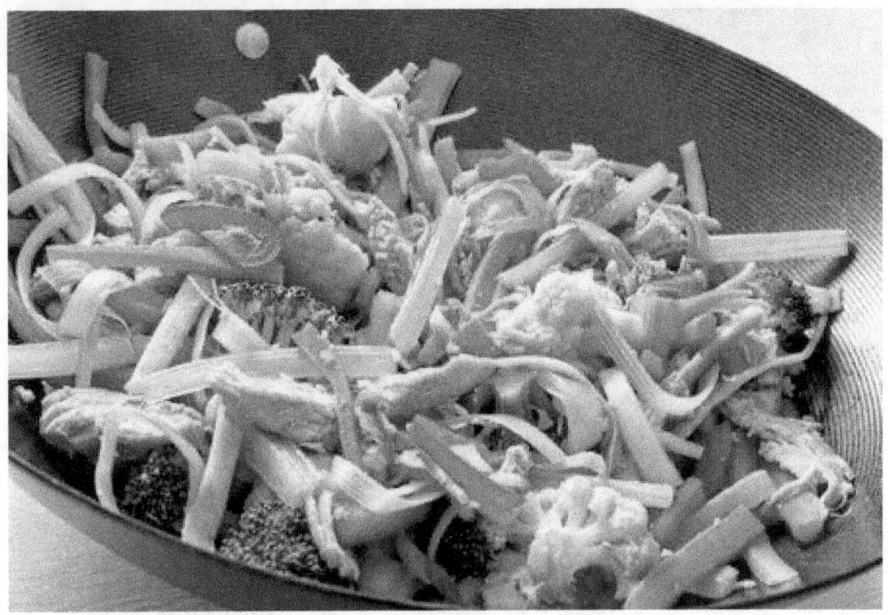

You may also want to add pieces of chicken to this stir Fry.

Fry a selection of all the available vegetables in your garden. These are going to include **florettes of cauliflower, spheres of broccoli, strips of carrot, roughly chopped leeks and onions, bean sprouts**, and any other vegetable.

You can either fry them in a Wok or if you want, you can fry them in 2 tablespoons oil, then simmer in about **half a pint of chicken stock and half a teaspoonful of soybean sauce** for ten minutes.

Garlic Prawns.

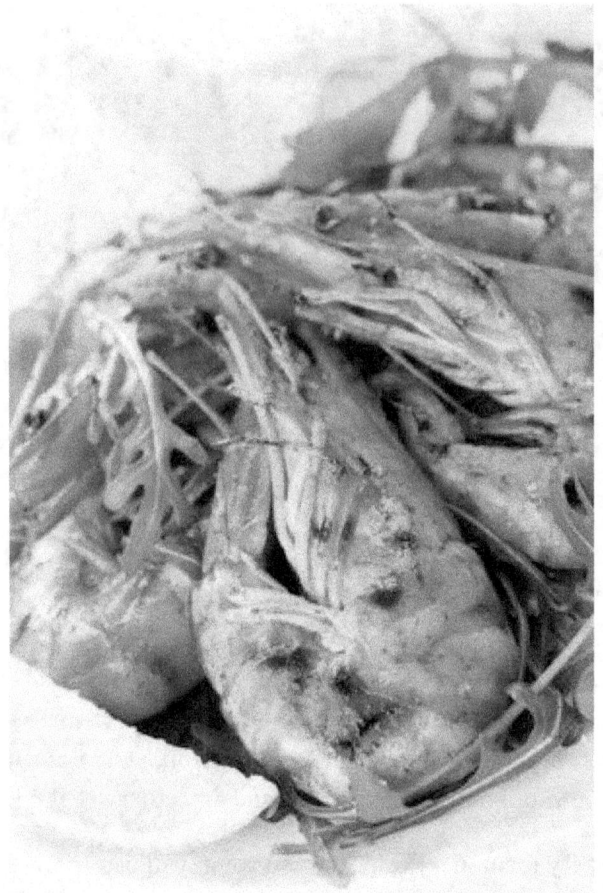

This is a delicacy, which can be found in huge quantities, on seaside stalls, especially in the coastal areas of Singapore, Malaysia, China and other areas where you can get prawns fresh from the sea.

Fry **half a pound of fresh prawns in a little oil with 2 crushed garlic cloves** for four – five minutes until cooked. Serve sprinkled with **soybean sauce and lemon.** Serves four people.

Duck in Orange Sauce

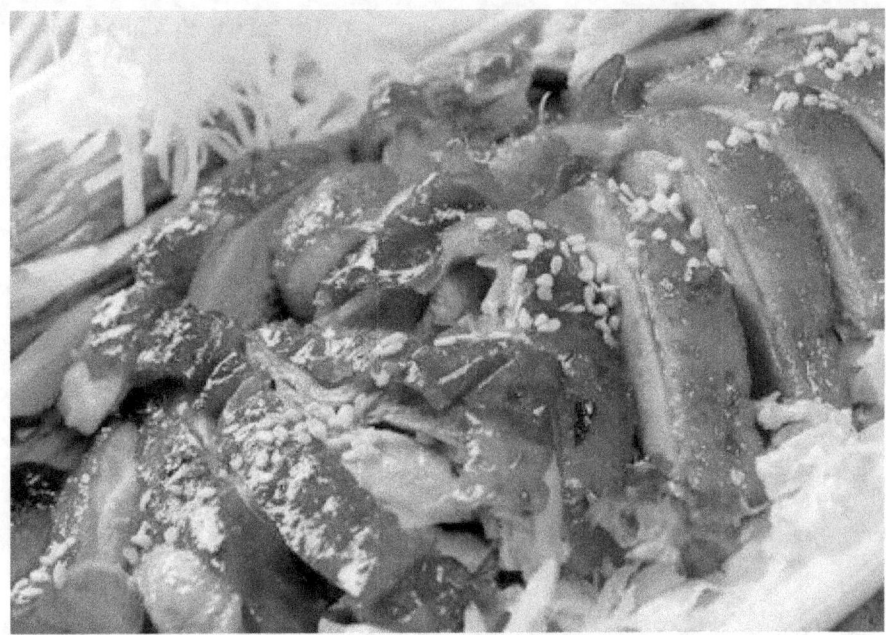

When I saw this on the menu and saw the exorbitant price being asked for duck in Orange sauce, I began to wonder why housewives did not make it more right at home. That is because many of these oriental dishes are considered to be luxury dishes in occidental kitchens. This is the idea being promulgated, that the ingredients are so exotic, rare to find, and expensive that they can only be eaten in five star restaurants by epicures and gourmets.

For duck in Orange sauce you need one small duck, roasted

For the sauce, you need 2 tablespoons full of soya sauce, 1 ½ teaspoons full of sugar, 6 tablespoons red wine, 6 tablespoons chicken stock, half a teaspoon chili sauce, half a red pepper, sliced juice of one orange, 1 ½ pieces of fresh root ginger, grated and two level teaspoons arrowroot.

Slice the duck. Put all the sauce ingredients in a pan, and simmer for two – three minutes. Add the sliced duck and let it heat for ten – fifteen minutes. Serve garnished with orange.

Beef Casserole

Casseroles in any form are extremely economical dishes, which you can just make, freeze, then reheat. This is going to serve four.

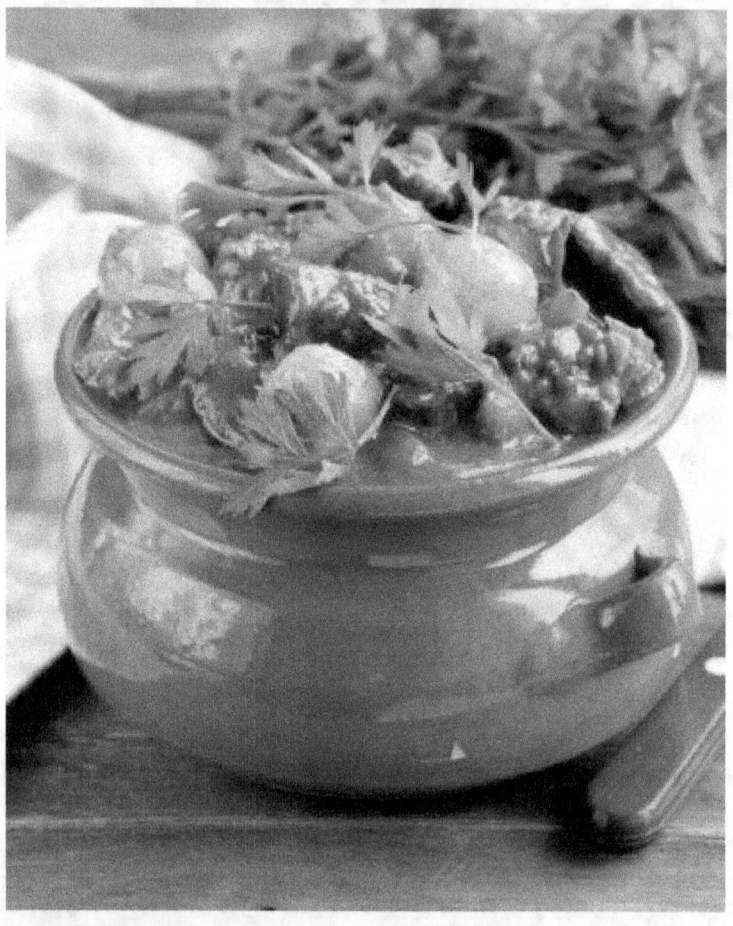

Half a pound of sirloin steak cubed
One onion, chopped
2 tablespoons oil
Half a pound of mushrooms, sliced
Three – four pieces canned bamboo shoots, sliced
One level teaspoons sugar
1 teaspoon vinegar
Half a pint of beef stock

1 tablespoon soy sauce

Fry the steak and onions in oil for a few minutes to seal the meat. Add the remaining ingredients and cook for about ten minutes or so, or until the meat is cooked through, then serve hot.

Fried Fish

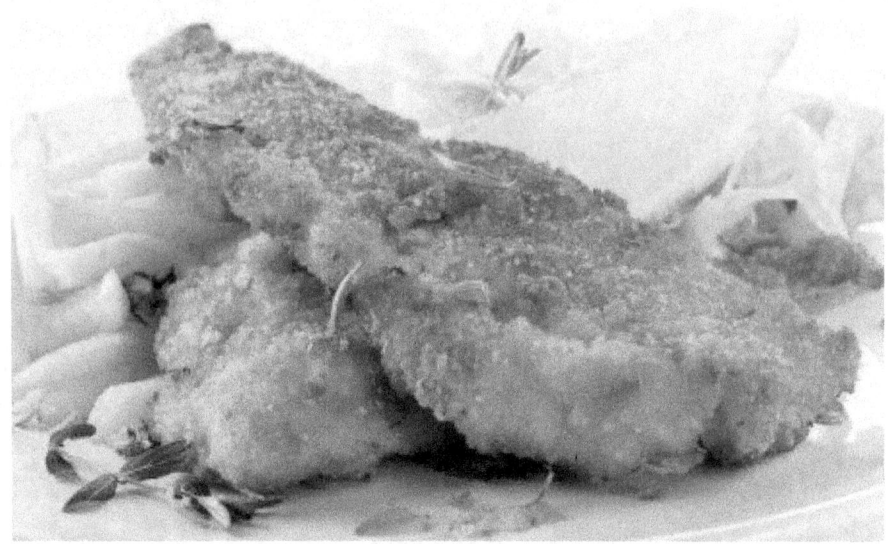

For four servings.

Sprinkle **half a pound of whiting fillets, cut into pieces with half a level teaspoon full of chili powder, the juice of half a lemon, and three crushed cloves of garlic.** Leave for thirty minutes. Dip in **egg batter, made up of one egg, 2 ounces plain flour, and 5 tablespoons full of milk**. Deep fry and serve with lemon.

Tandoori Chicken

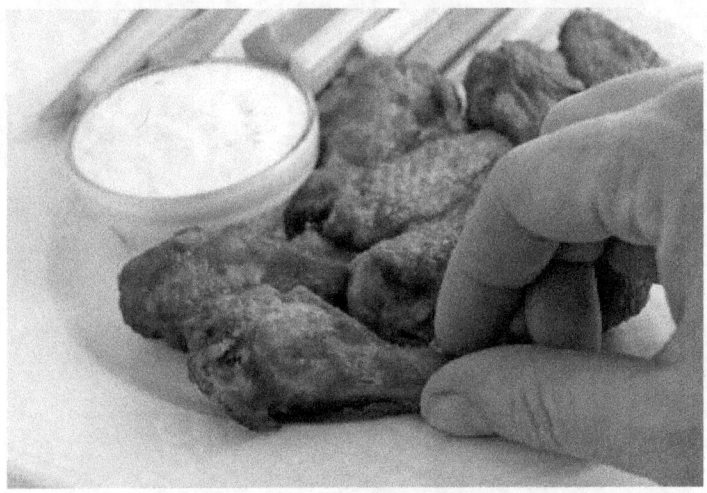

Traditional tandoori chicken is normally made in a clay oven called a tandoor. This is going to serve four people.

Mix **half a pint of natural yogurt with two level teaspoons tandoori spice mixture, one crushed clove of garlic, and the juice of half a lemon.** Rub this into **four well slashed chicken joints** and roast or grill until they are cooked.

Garnished with slices of onion and serve with 6 ounces of boiled rice, which has been cooked with lemon juice and a pinch of turmeric.

Okra in Tomato Sauce

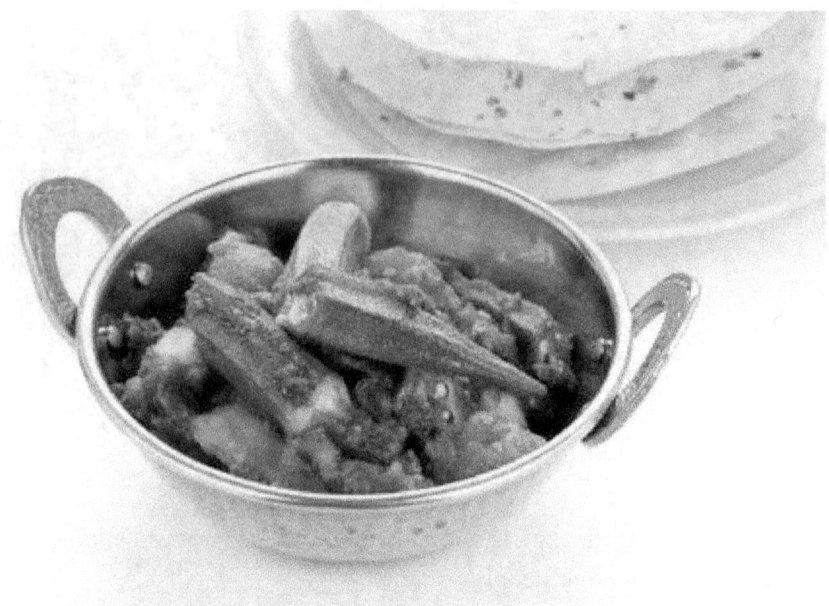

This traditional dish shown above is made by not slicing the okra in small pieces, but cutting the full vegetables with narrow slices in which one puts in a mixture of salt, dried herbs, spices and red chili pepper to taste.

Serves four.

Half a pound of okra, topped and kept whole.
One large onion, very coarsely chopped
Two cloves of garlic, crushed
1 ounce of butter.
2 tablespoons oil
One green chili, deseeded and finely chopped
1 teaspoon coarsely ground coriander seeds.
Good pinch of turmeric.
One level teaspoon chopped mint.
Six large tomatoes.

Fry the okra, onion and garlic in the butter and oil for a few minutes, then add the remaining ingredients. Simmer, covered, for twenty – thirty minutes. This is normally served with boiled rice, or with fresh bread.

Kofta Curry

Kofta means minced meat balls.

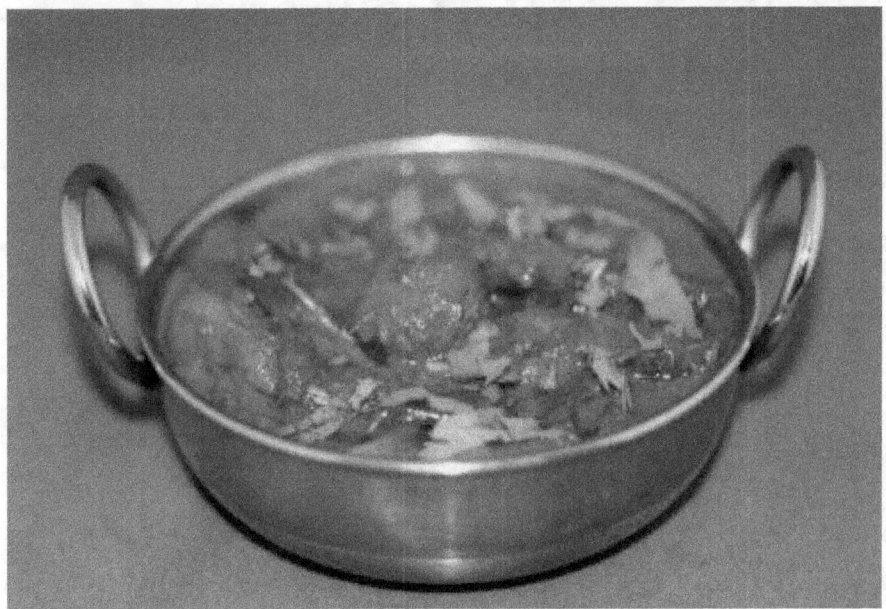

Four servings. I used this recipe to make hamburger patties, instead of curries, and they turned up really delicious.

Half a pound of minced meat – you can use hamburger meat. You can also use half a pound of minced beef, if it comes cheaper.
Half a pound of onions, half grated and the remainder coarsely chopped
Two cloves of garlic, crushed
Two yolks of eggs.
One level teaspoon cumin seeds
1 ounce fresh bread crumbs
Herbs and spices of your choice for seasoning. Use parsley, rosemary, sage, thyme, basil, garlic salt, rock salt, and whatever else you have in your herb cabinet.
Oil for deep frying
2 ounces of butter.
1 inch piece of fresh root ginger, peeled and finely chopped
One level teaspoons full of salt.

Half a level teaspoon each of chili powder, ground black pepper, garam masala powder, turmeric, paprika, pepper

Half a pint of natural yogurt.

Half a pint of beef stock or chicken stock

Mix the beef with the grated onions, egg yolk, garlic, cumin, bread crumbs and seasoning herbs. Form this mixture into bite sized balls.

Deep fry in oil until they are cooked.

Fry the chopped onions in the butter until lightly golden. Fry the ginger, add spices and salt and stir in the stock. Simmer ten minutes before adding the meatballs and yogurt.

Boil, then simmer for another ten minutes to get a rich, delicious curry, stirring carefully so that the meat balls do not break.

Sukiyaki

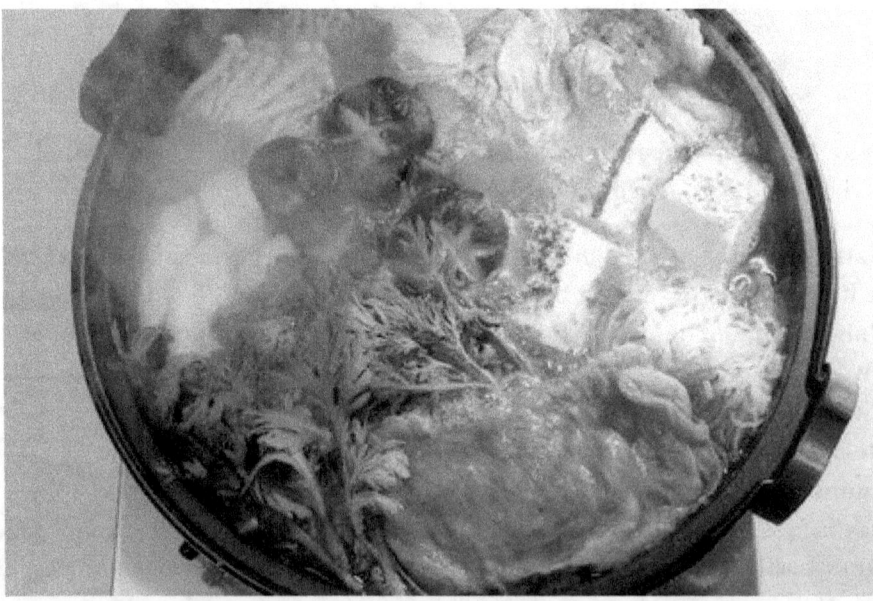

Japanese dishes have excellent nutritional value, as well as texture, color, and flavor. So when you are frying these ingredients in a wok, the idea is put all the ingredients together in a wok and stir fry at a high heat moving the utensil over the fire, often so that the heat can go all the vegetables and the meat evenly.

I asked a Japanese friend if sukiyaki was a traditional Japanese dish. Because I knew that chicken chow mein and chicken chopsuey are definitely not traditional Chinese dishes. They were thought up by a Chinese chef in Singapore during the Second World War to feed hungry American troops. And now they are an integral part of restaurant or street food cuisine all over the world!

She told me that it was a popular food – not exactly traditional, but a healthy part of Japanese cuisine

Sukiyaki is made by rolling about ten – 12 ounces of well beaten sirloin steak into small rolls. Fry them in 2 tablespoons full of oil in a wok or frying pan until they begin to brown. Add eight spring onions, chopped into short lengths, one large green pepper sliced, four carrots, sliced, one Chinese cabbage, sliced into 2 inch sections, 8 ounce can of drained sliced bamboo shoots, four pieces of bean curd, 2 ounces of any thin noodles – try Saifun stirfry noodles – steep them in hot water for three minutes and then drain – 6 ounces fresh bean sprouts and eight mushrooms.

Add these vegetables in the wok in this order so that the harder vegetables can cook longer.

Stir with fork or with chopsticks.

Mix one level teaspoons full of sugar, with half a pint of chicken stock and one – 3 tablespoons full of Japanese soy sauce, depending on your taste.

Stir into the wok or pan and simmer three – four minutes.

Serve mixed with beaten egg in individual bowls with boiled rice.

Managing Your Tomato Harvest

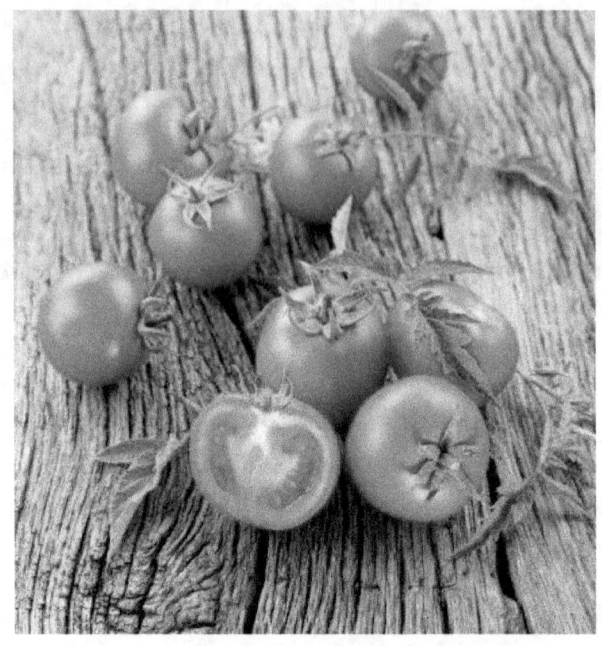

If you have a really good tomato harvest, why not make lots of tomato sauce. For that you need **1 ounce butter, one large onion, chopped, 2 pounds skinned tomatoes, one level teaspoon full brown sugar, fresh basil and sage, salt and pepper.** This is going to make half a pint – ¾ pint of tomato sauce, depending on your harvest and the size of the tomatoes.

Melt the butter and fry the onion until it is soft. Add the chopped tomatoes, sugars, herbs and seasoning. Simmer gently for about one hour. Instead of putting the sauce into bottles, I normally freeze them in small bags are in ice cube trays. And I slip out the amount I need and defreeze a cube or two before adding to my dish.

Excellent sauce addition to thicken gravies and curries.

Traditional Onion Bread

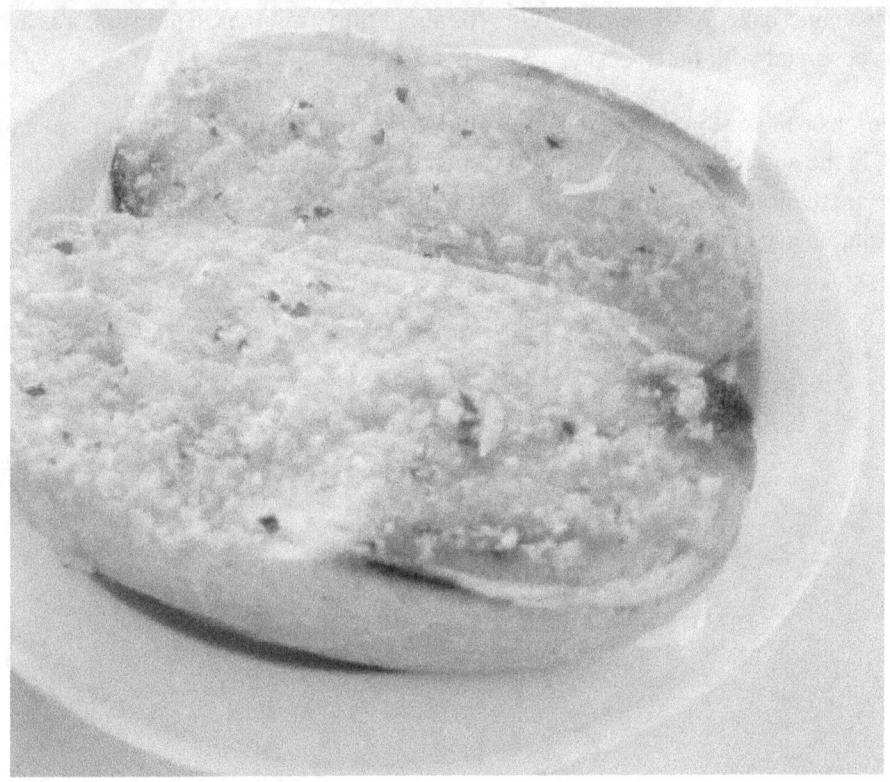

Onion and garlic bread is traditional breakfast fare in many European countries.

8 to 10 people can be fed well on this traditional onion bread, which is made up of **1 ounce fresh yeast or half an ounce of dried yeast, half a teaspoonful of sugar, 1 pound of plain flour, sieved, one pinch of salt, half a pound of onions, sliced, butter or oil for frying, seasoning, one teaspoonful of herbs.**

Cream the fresh yeast and sugar, or mix the dry yeast with sugar and half a pint of lukewarm water and leave until the mixture turns frothy.

Mix the yeast into flour, with salt and sufficient extra liquid – about half a pint – to give a firm, pliable dough. Knead well, and leave to double.

Knead again, till it reaches its original size. This is called knocking back. Spread over base of greased ovenproof dish. Fry onions in fat and spread over dough. Season and bake, Mark seven – 425° for about thirty minutes. Cut in squares and serve, spread with butter.

Onions can be stored in strings. Carefully remove from the ground and leave to dry in the sun for a few days – or in a shed or garage, if the weather is wet. Once dry, tie them by their foliage in long strands or bunches of weight. Hang them in a suitable dry place for the winter.

Conclusion

In the USA, the authorities for Health Education have been planning a vast amount of money to advertise to men, women and children the dangers of overeating. That kind of message is not new – Americans have been urged to ease up on the quantity and type of food they have got used to eating for years.

Calorie counting is not everything – one should eat for the sheer pleasure of sampling tastes and textures, because they matter more. Now, if you have a wider choice of exciting yet healthy ways of cooking and presenting familiar foods that one tended to serve in the same old way for years in the past, would not you take the choice to experiment?

This book is full of tips and techniques with ideas, which you would want to utilize when you are making tasty meals, within a budget.

Buy oil in solid form – it looks like lard, but it is made from palm oil. There is no need to refrigerate – once used, pour it into a basin and it is going to solidify at room temperature.

The price for this solid oil is more economical, when you compare it with other files in the market.

If your cholesterol plungers, yet reluctant to give up the flavor of butter, then try a new mix called Gold. That is, if you have it on your market shelves. Do not mix it up with Kerry Gold, which is pure Irish butter. Gold is a blend of butter, oil and vegetable fats. You can spread this from the fridge and it has just over half as many calories as butter.

You can also make something special out of simple ice cream, mousse and blancmange by squirting a bit of dessert topping on top. This is made by mixing some topping with a little jam or brandy or just stirring into partially frozen ice cream to make a homemade ripple ice.

The flavors of the East in the form of spices are extremely delicious ingredients to add a zing factor to your dishes. Jars of exotic spices may look like an expensive buy, but many of them keep more or less indefinitely, and they also make clever cooking effortless.

Live Long and Prosper!

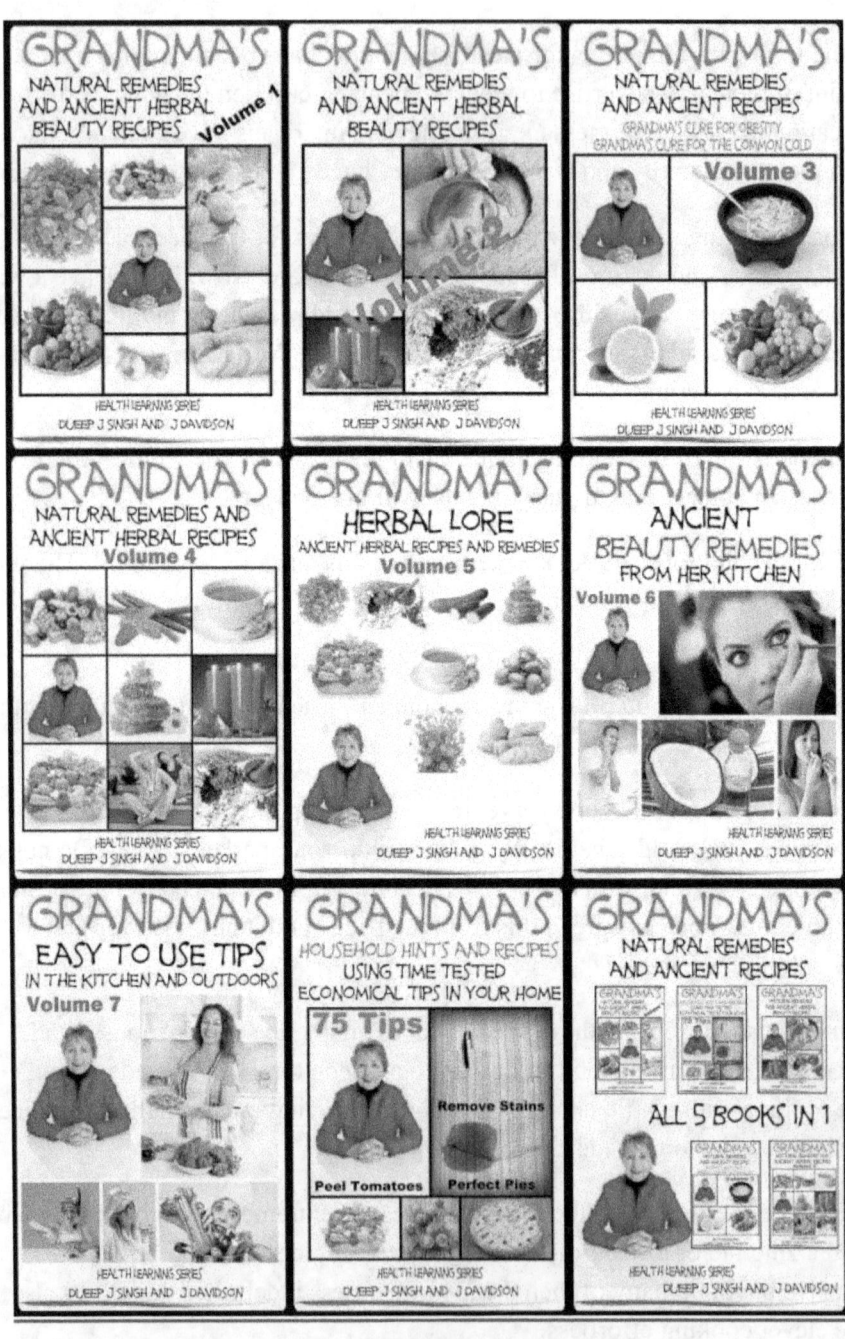

Author Bio

Dueep Jyot Singh is a Management and IT Professional who managed to gather Postgraduate qualifications in Management and English and Degrees in Science, French and Education while pursuing different enjoyable career options like being an hospital administrator, IT,SEO and HRD Database Manager/ trainer, movie , radio and TV scriptwriter, theatre artiste and public speaker, lecturer in French, Marketing and Advertising, ex-Editor of Hearts On Fire (now known as Solstice) Books Missouri USA, advice columnist and cartoonist, publisher and Aviation School trainer, ex- moderator on Medico.in, banker, student councilor ,travelogue writer ... among other things!

One fine morning, she decided that she had enough of killing herself by Degrees and went back to her first love -- writing. It's more enjoyable! She already has 48 published academic and 14 fiction- in- different- genre books under her belt.

When she is not designing websites or making Graphic design illustrations for clients , she is browsing through old bookshops hunting for treasures, of which she has an enviable collection – including R.L. Stevenson, O.Henry, Dornford Yates, Maurice Walsh, De Maupassant, Victor Hugo, Sapper, C.N. Williamson, "Bartimeus" and the crown of her collection- Dickens "The Old Curiosity Shop," and so on... Just call her "Renaissance Woman") - collecting herbal remedies, acting like Universal Helping Hand/Agony Aunt, or escaping to her dear mountains for a bit of exploring, collecting herbs and plants and trekking.

1. Amazon.com
2. Barnes and Noble
3. Itunes
4. Kobo
5. Smashwords
6. Google Play Books

Check out some of the other JD-Biz Publishing books

Gardening Series on Amazon

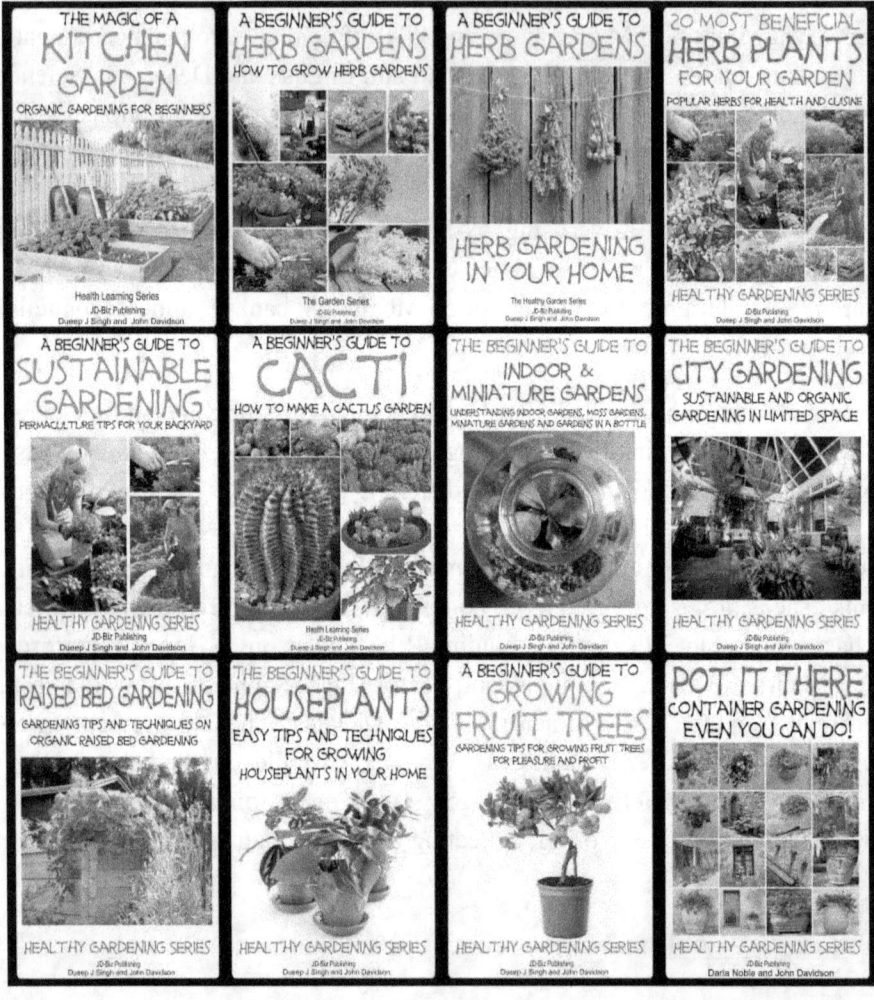

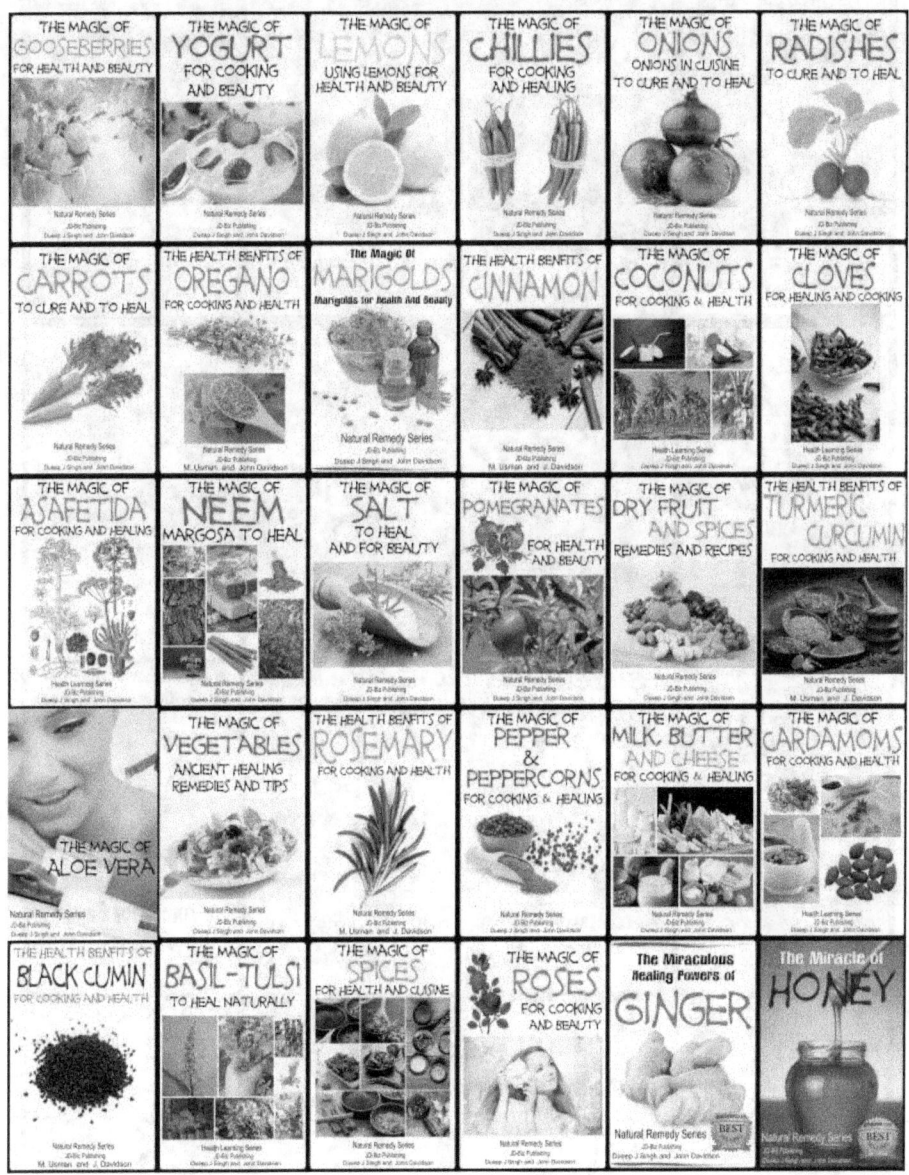

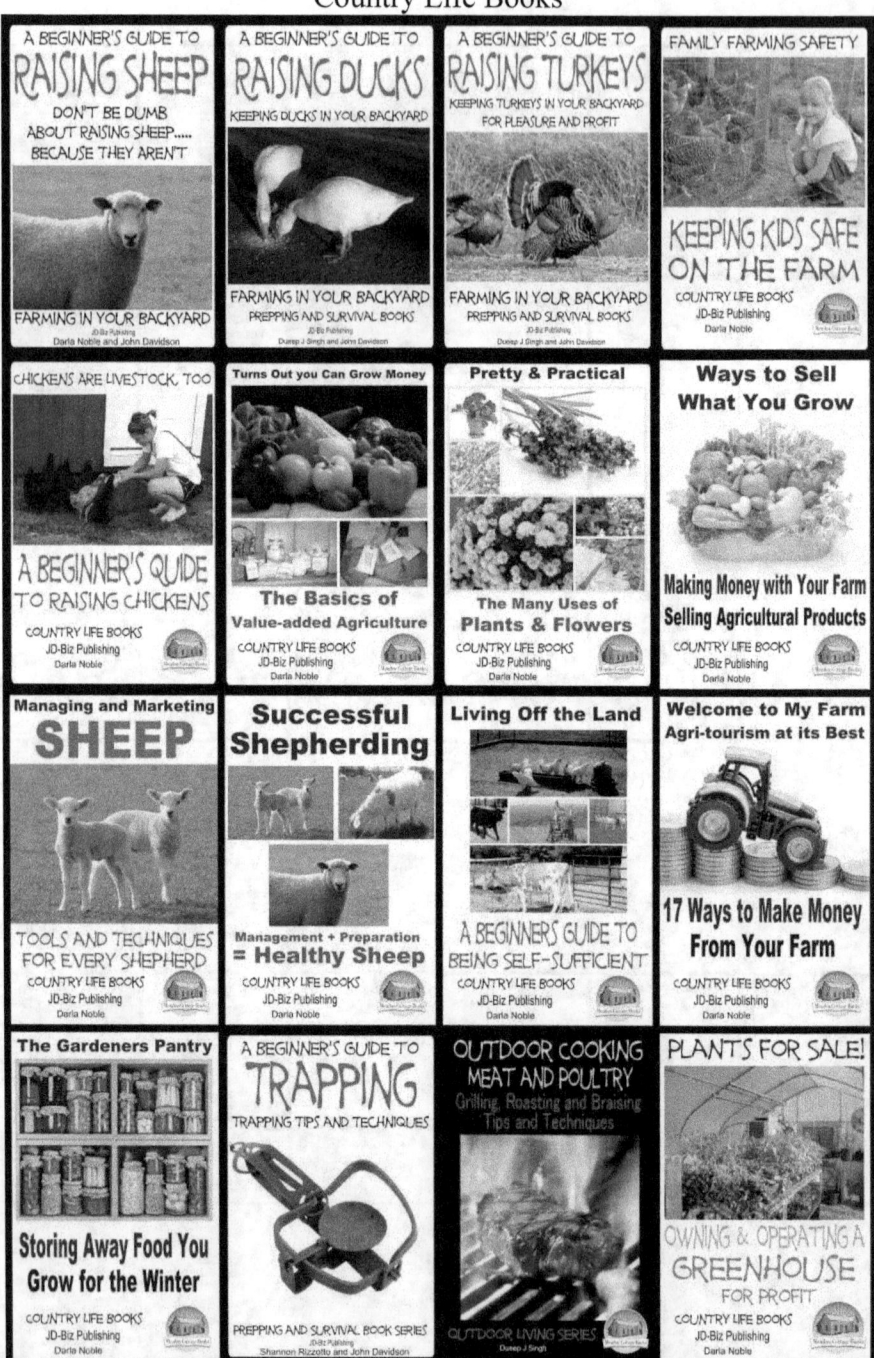

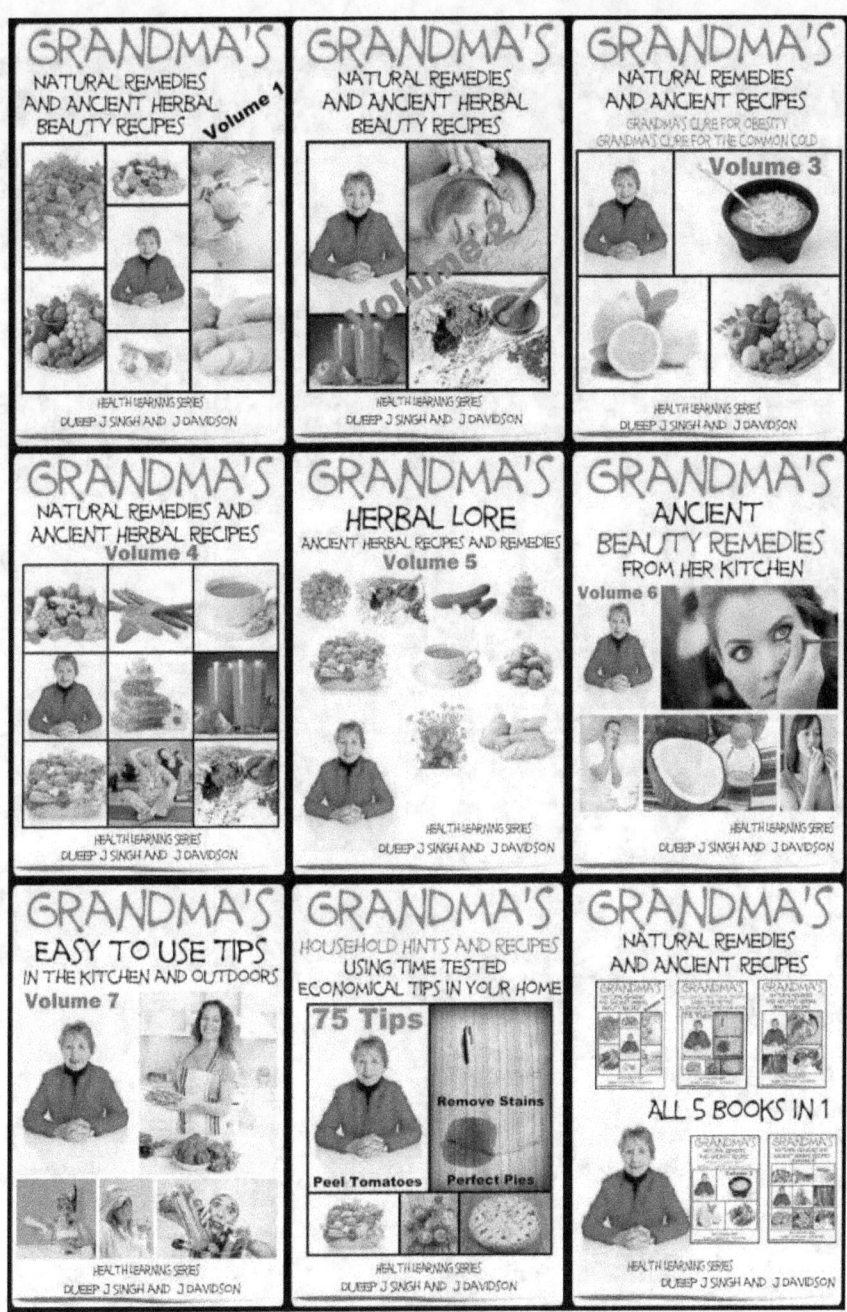

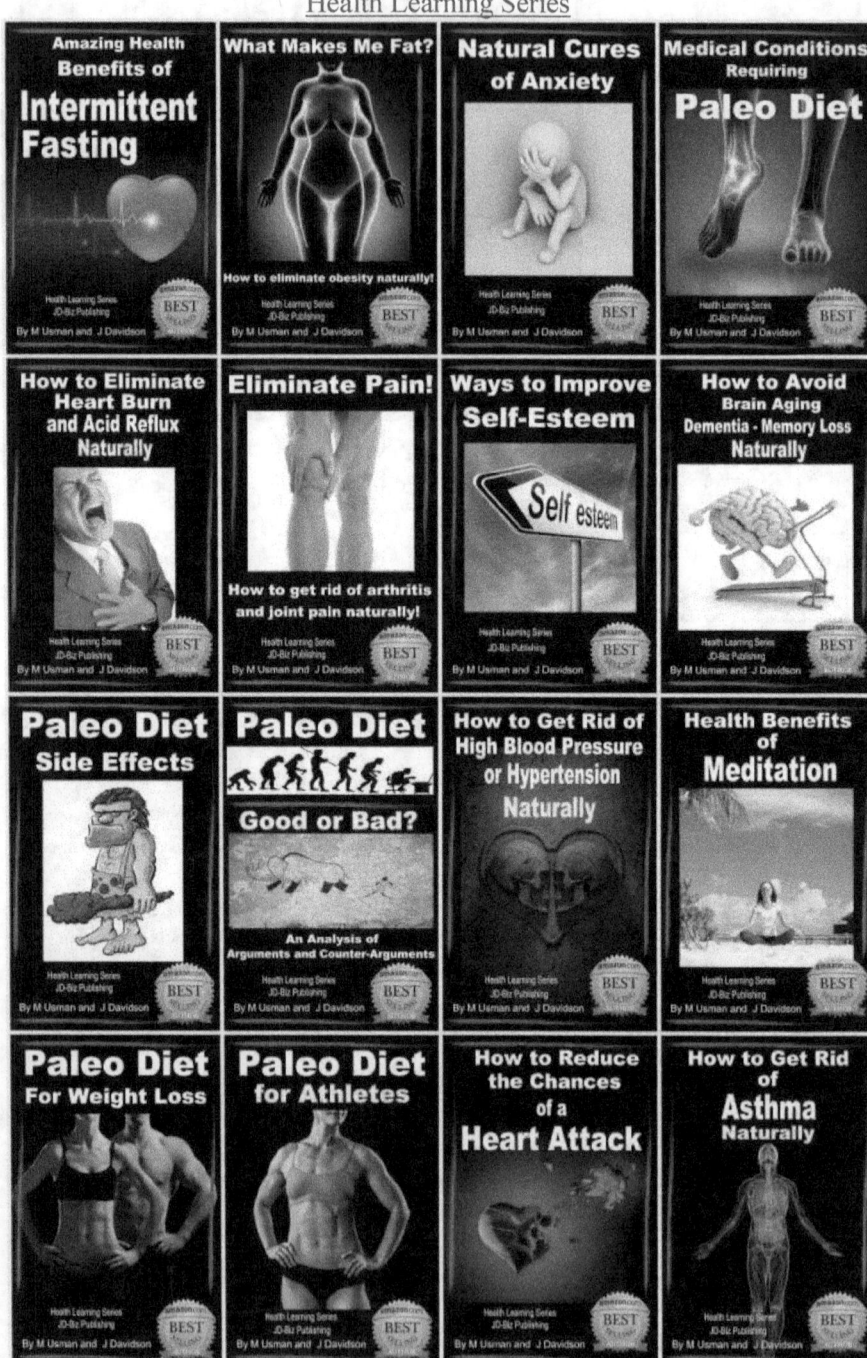

Amazing Animal Book Series

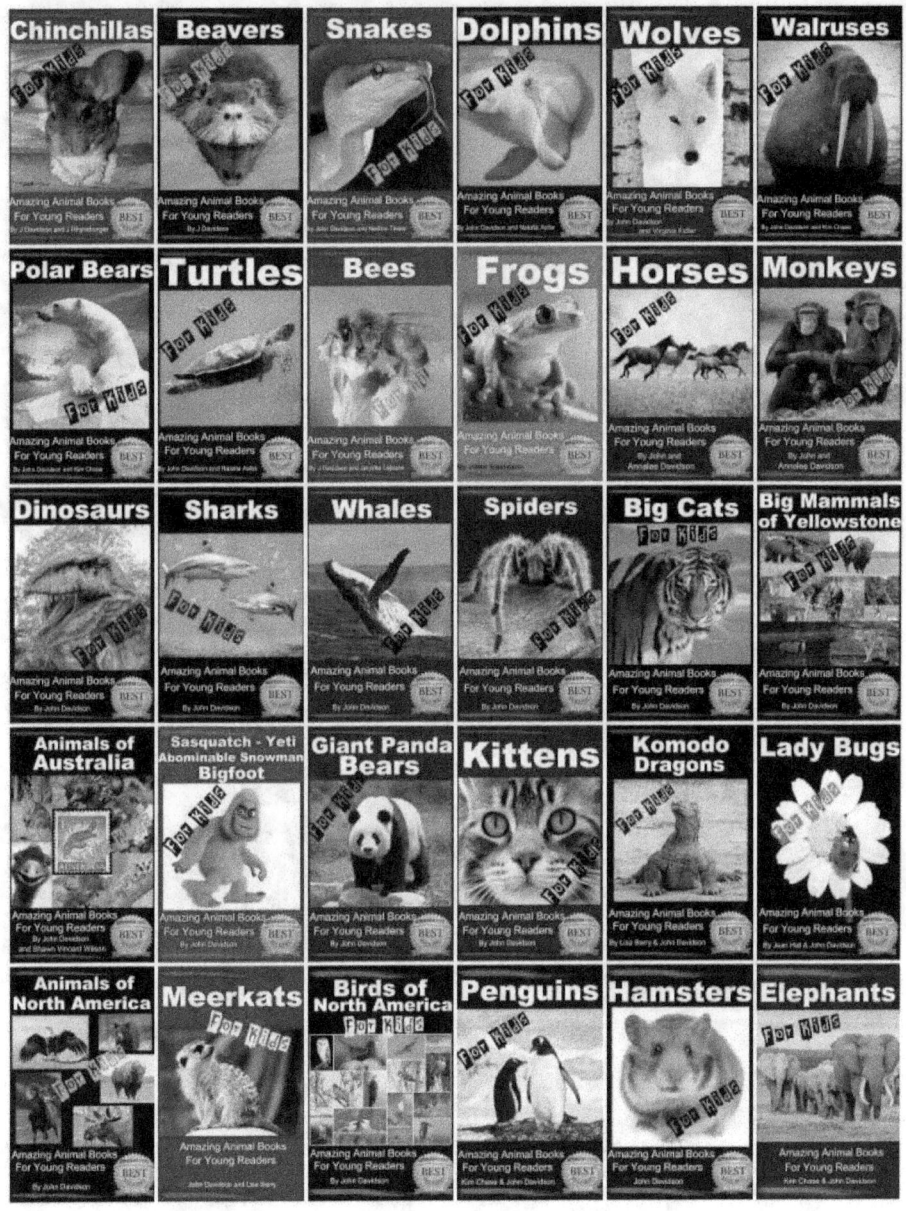

Learn To Draw Series

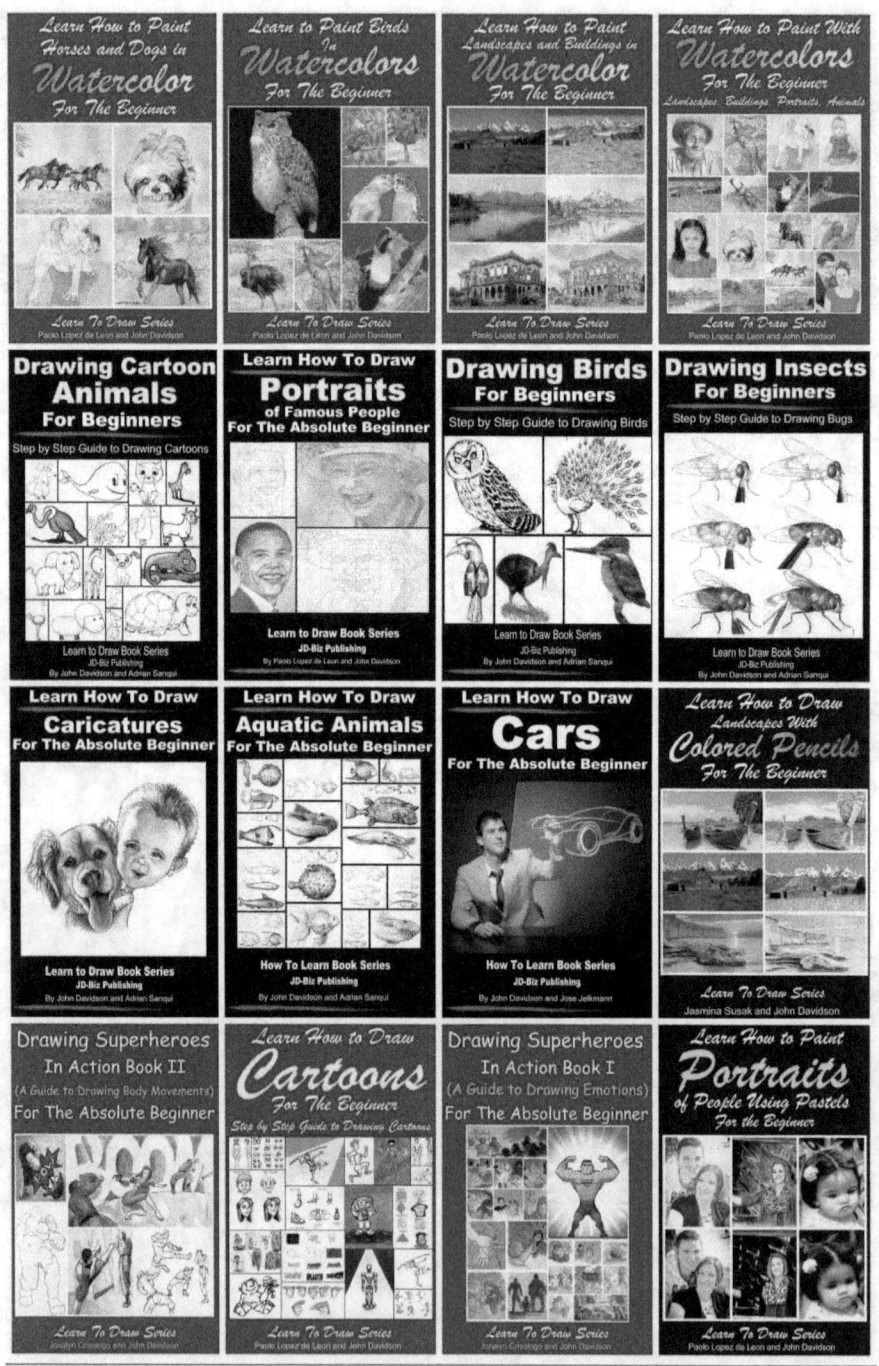

How to Build and Plan Books

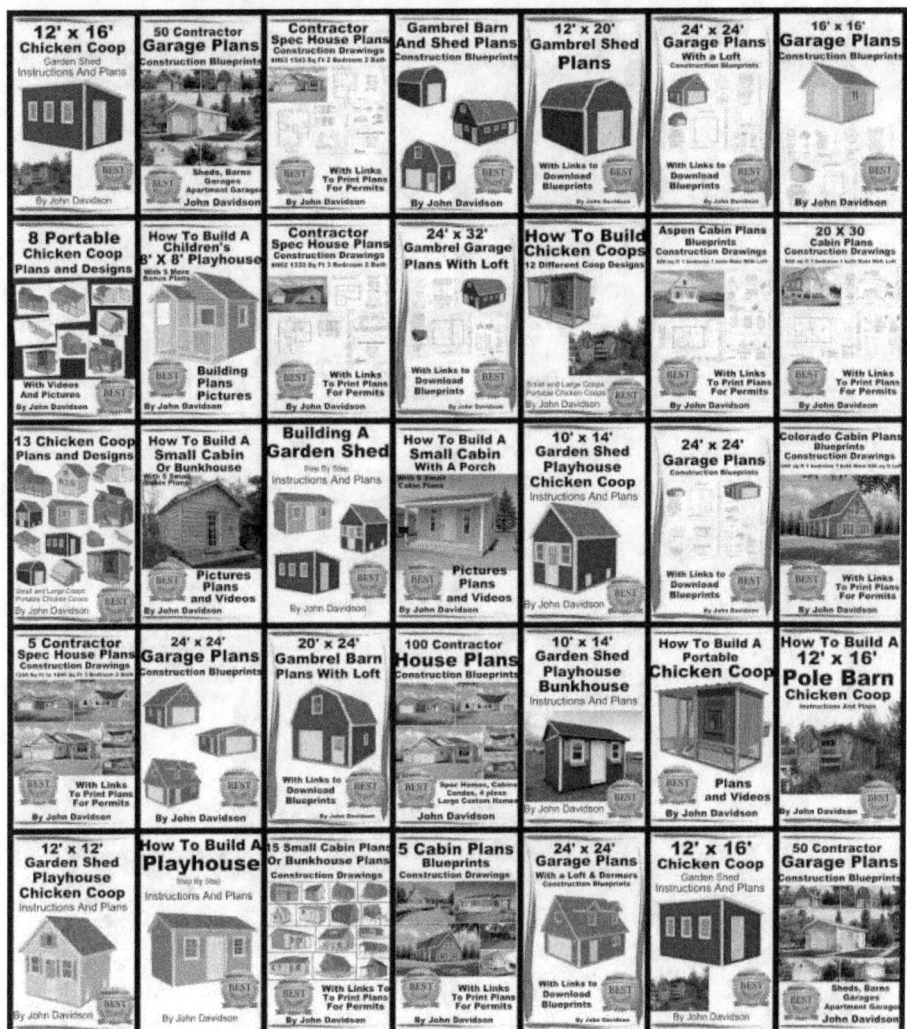

Entrepreneur Book Series

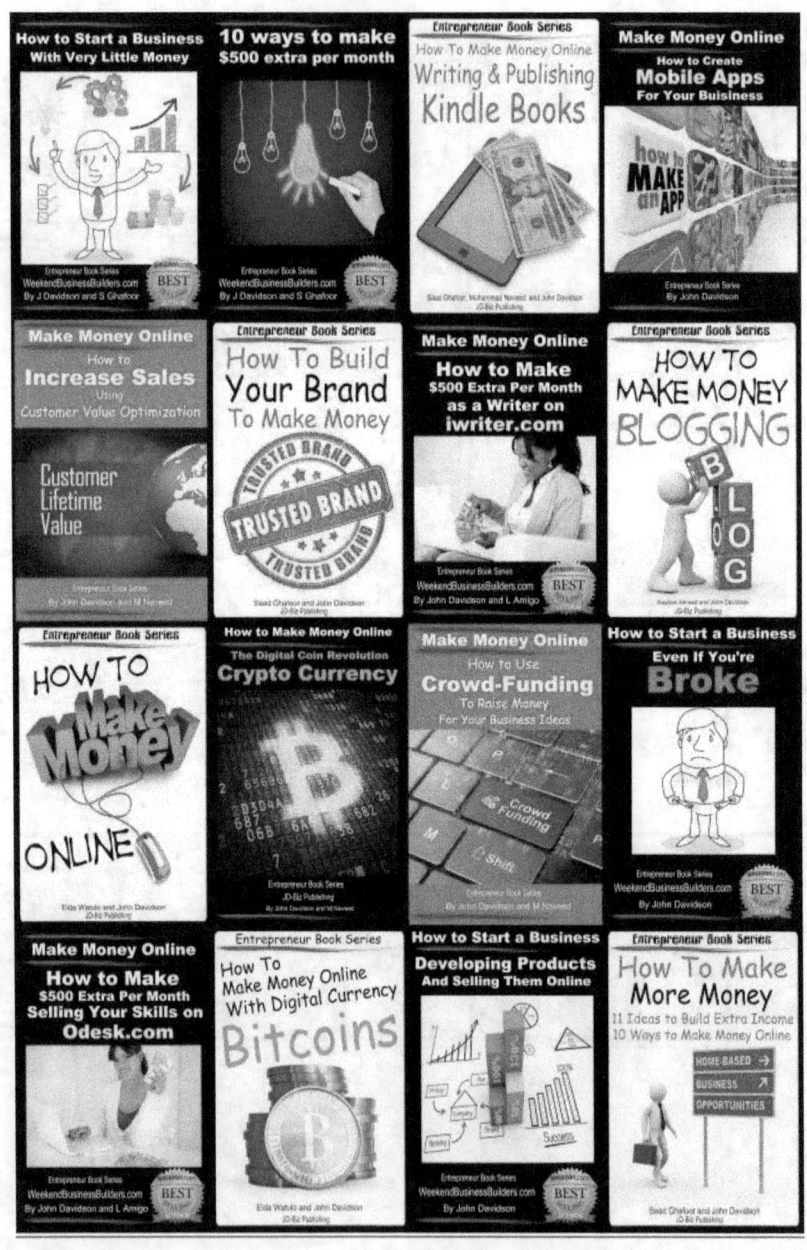

Publisher

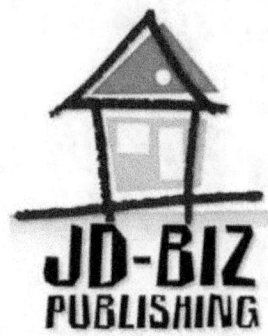

JD-Biz Corp

P O Box 374

Mendon, Utah 84325

http://www.jd-biz.com/

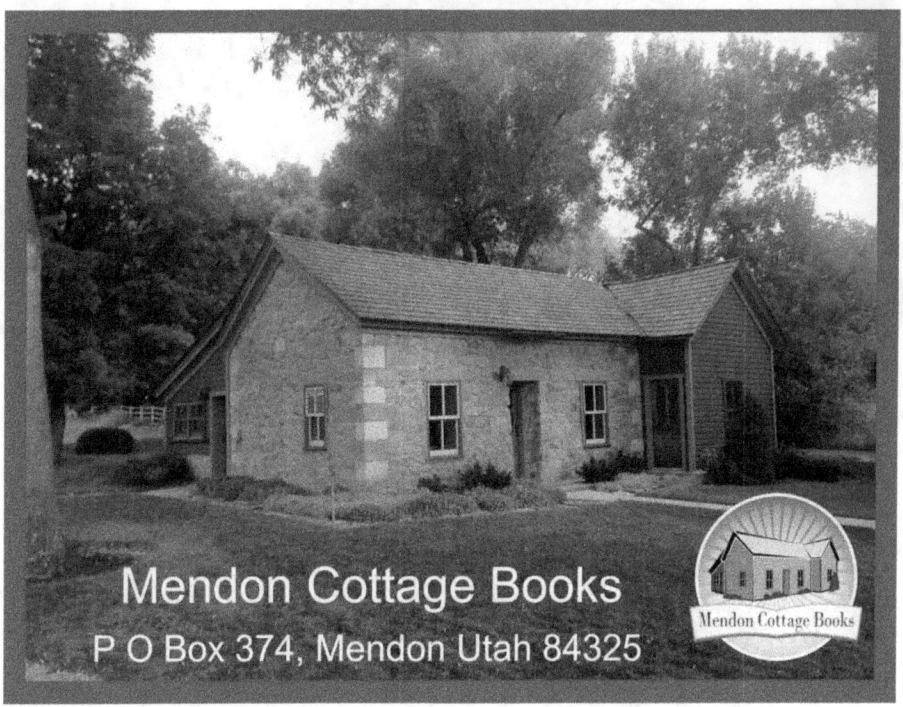

www.ingramcontent.com/pod-product-compliance
Lightning Source LLC
Chambersburg PA
CBHW060649290526
45793CB00001B/469